MINDFULNESS ACTIVITIES
FOR ADULTS

MINDFULNESS ACTIVITIES for adults

50 Simple Exercises to Relax, Stay Present, and Find Peace

MATTHEW REZAC, MPS, ACC

ROCKRIDGE
PRESS

To Emma, Megan, Annie, and Kate.
Thank you for helping me learn to be
openhearted, even during stressful times.

Interior and Cover Designer: Elizabeth Zuhl
Art Producer: Meg Baggott
Editor: Annie Choi
Production Manager: Holly Haydash

Author photo courtesy of Cindy McAndrew/Brightside Creative

Paperback ISBN: 978-1-63807-053-5 | eBook ISBN: 978-1-63807-580-6
R0

Contents

Introduction

Welcome to *Mindfulness Activities for Adults*, a collection of 50 simple, engaging activities designed to support your mindfulness practice—no matter where you are on your journey.

My name is Matt Rezac, and I am a mindfulness-based life coach. I teach the Art of Engaged Mindfulness at the Mindfulness Coaching School, which is about practicing mindfulness in everyday life.

Mindfulness can seem serious and intimidating, but it actually helps us be more spontaneous, present, and lighthearted. The goal of this book is to make mindfulness feel natural—and even fun—using simple activities that can help you experience more peace and joy.

You can use this book however you like, but it can work well:

◆ For individual practice or with family and friends.

◆ As a 50-day mindfulness "challenge."

◆ As a weekly practice prompt.

◆ Whenever you need a grounding moment of peace.

I hope this book helps you use mindfulness to improve life each day. Now, let's look at a few mindfulness basics and how this book is organized.

What Is Mindfulness?

There are many definitions of mindfulness. Perhaps the most famous is from Jon Kabat-Zinn, the developer of mindfulness-based stress reduction (MBSR). In his January 2017 interview in *Mindful* magazine, he describes mindfulness as "paying attention, on purpose, in the present moment, non-judgmentally." Here's another good way to think about mindfulness:

Who: Mindfulness begins with you and your perception. It often leads to insights about your relationships with others.

What: Mindfulness is a practice of acceptance. It's not ignoring what needs to change but radically accepting the current reality as a starting place.

When: Mindfulness happens now, in the present moment.

Where: Mindfulness happens here, wherever you are.

How: Mindfulness accesses a basic awareness that is always available to you.

Why: There are many reasons to practice mindfulness, including stress reduction, insight, performance, and better relationships.

Being mindful is actually very simple, but our default is to practice "non-mindfulness." Breaking that habit is the challenge.

How Mindfulness Works

The human brain is amazing. It's home to 100 billion neurons, each connected to up to 15,000 other neurons through electrical signals called synapses. Everything we experience correlates to synapses firing between neurons across the brain.

The strongest neural connections link to our most frequent experiences. Some are vital, like breathing and heart functioning. Strong neural connections can also form around unhealthy habits like obsessive worrying or addictive behaviors. Mindfulness helps bring awareness to our habitual actions and create opportunities to make new choices. By practicing mindfulness, we can gradually weaken strong neural connections that correlate with bad habits. Yes, mindfulness literally changes our brains!

Mindfulness also changes our bodies. It activates the parasympathetic nervous system, which helps calm us by lowering our heart rate, blood pressure, muscle tension, and respiratory rate.

Research has shown that mindfulness may result in the following benefits:

♦ Decreased anxiety and depression

♦ Improved immune function

♦ Increased clarity and focus

♦ A more resilient brain

♦ Improved self-confidence

♦ Improved mood and sleep

Mindfulness is not a cure-all, however. If you have history of trauma, you may want to explore trauma-sensitive mindfulness techniques as you begin or deepen your practice.

How to Use This Book

Many activities in this book are similar to traditional mindfulness exercises but are designed to be as engaging as possible. The goal is to help you relax and have fun. For example, we might practice breathing meditation by imagining ourselves at the beach, which is a relatable and spontaneous way to relax. Best of all, you don't need much time, special tools, or previous experience to play.

The activities are divided into the following five topics:

Breath. Our breath is a portable teacher. No matter where we are or what we're doing, the breath can return us to the present moment. Cultivating awareness of the breath is often the foundational step in developing mindful awareness.

Mind. Our minds work hard, trying to help us by making sense of the world. But often they become "monkey minds," filled with chattering, anxious thoughts. Mindfulness helps us abide in awareness instead of the mind's latest worries.

Body. Our bodies send us powerful, subtle signals. Through mindfulness, we gain valuable information to support our own well-being.

Connection. We are interconnected with all things, yet we can feel lonely, isolated, and pressured to be self-dependent. Mindfulness helps us see our interconnection and act in ways that support healthy relationships.

Joy. Mindfulness brings joy! Sometimes it looks like a solemn, pensive undertaking, but you won't find that here. We're going for silly grins, open hearts, and savoring the aliveness found in any moment.

While these topics build on one another, there's no right or wrong way to use this book. Have fun with it! Dive in and skip around however you like.

ICONS

Before each activity, you will see the number of players, time required, and any supplies you might need. In addition, each activity is marked with an icon that tells you which of the following themes it fits into:

 Creativity. These involve a creative activity, like drawing, coloring, or simple movements.

 Everyday. This category relates to daily tasks, such as driving or taking care of your to-do list.

 Nature. Use nature activities to get outdoors or interact with nature.

 Quick. These can be done in five minutes or less.

Creating a Practice

Enjoying and benefiting from this book can be as simple as choosing an activity and playing it. However, if you want to dive more deeply into mindfulness and start an intentional, ongoing mindfulness practice, here is some concrete advice on how to get started:

Making time. Many of us feel chronically out of time, but mindfulness can happen whenever it works best for you! Practicing at the same time each day can help build momentum. Once you've established a routine, you may notice it's easier to find time. Start by practicing for one to five minutes, three to five times per day.

Creating space. It helps to create a designated place in a quiet corner for your practice. It can include things like a meditation cushion, candles, and inspiring quotes or photos. This can motivate you to practice regularly, but it is not necessary. Mindfulness practice can happen anywhere you create alert awareness.

Setting intentions. Mindfulness can help you clarify intentions and direct your awareness toward activities that support your well-being. What do you hope to manifest in your life? What gentle actions might nudge you toward the future you want? I recommend seeking out teachers to help guide you in setting intentions (online videos are great resources for this).

Building consistency. Like brushing your teeth, the benefits of mindfulness accrue through regular practice. A single mindfulness exercise can provide a quick, temporary state of relaxation. Making that temporary experience a lasting state requires consistency. Loch Kelly of the Nondual Mindfulness Institute emphasizes "small glimpses, many times" (such as five to seven shorter practices per day) as a strategy to develop consistency.

Reflecting. We are constantly stimulated to take action, whether by social media, our boss, a load of unfolded laundry, or any number of factors. Flinging ourselves from action to action, we miss opportunities to rest, learn, and grow. Uninterrupted reflection (like journaling, conversation, or alone time) complements mindfulness to provide positive, lasting benefits.

BREATH

YOUR BEAUTIFUL BREATH

PLAYER: 1 | **TIME:** 5 MINUTES

The breath is a handy tool for cultivating mindfulness. You take it with you wherever you go. It provides an always present, repeating cycle that's perfect for anchoring awareness: inhale, pause, exhale, pause. Yet no two breaths are exactly alike. Sometimes, the breath is choppy and shallow. Other times, it is deep and drawn out. Through challenges and calm, we keep moving forward, just like the breath. This activity cultivates awareness of your simple, life-giving, beautiful breath.

---

1. Find a comfortable, alert position with your eyes open or closed.

2. Bring awareness to your breath. Notice where and when you are first aware of the breath cycle. Most of us might point to the nostrils, during inhalation, as the "starting point" of the breath cycle. But is this really where and when the breath begins?

3. Now bring more awareness to the air going in and out at your nostrils. How much sensation can you experience there? Explore these questions:

- ◆ How fast is the air moving?

- ◆ What temperature is the air?

- ◆ How is the temperature different between when you exhale and inhale?

- ◆ Where on your nostrils can you first feel the air?

- ◆ Where inside your nostrils does the sensation seem to end?

4. Next, bring your awareness to the top of your throat, just behind your mouth. What does the breath feel like at this point in its journey?

5. Now move your awareness to the breath as it moves in and out of your throat between the head and body. During the pause between inhale and exhale, does the breath remain inside your throat?

6. Next, shift awareness to the breath in your chest. Can you feel your lungs and rib cage expanding and contracting? How would you describe the quantity of air that fills your lungs?

7. Finally, notice the breath at your diaphragm and into your belly. How deep does your breath go? Can you bring more air into the deepest part of the belly?

A STORM NEVER HURT THE SKY.

BREATHING THE OCEAN

With each breath, we can connect with nature. We inhale oxygen provided by nature and offer carbon dioxide back when we exhale. Nature can be as foreboding as tornadoes and as sublime as a snowy landscape. Here we are, always breathing it in, but we normally don't notice that our own breath creates a moment-to-moment connection to our surroundings. In this activity, you will use mindfulness and imagination to reconnect with the world around you.

---

1. Find a comfortable, alert position either seated or lying down.

2. Close your eyes and focus on your breath. Notice where it is in its cycle: inhaling, exhaling, or paused between. (If you're holding your breath, let it flow!)

3. Watch your breath go through its cycle a few times. Just feel the experience of your body breathing.

4. Now imagine yourself on a beach watching the water come and go. Create an image in your mind's eye of the water's edge receding and advancing at the shore. It is gentle and powerful.

5. When you're ready, on the next inhalation, imagine a small ocean wave building momentum toward the beach. Connect the sound of the air entering your lungs with the sound of the water moving closer to the shoreline. Time the scene in your imagination so it seems like your inhalation is pulling the water onto the shore.

6. At the top of your breath, imagine the wave making its farthest reach onto the beach. See the water like a sheet pulled along the top of the sand. Hear the hypnotic whoosh of its crest.

7. While you exhale, imagine the water rolling back toward the ocean. Notice how it seems to dissipate, relax, and release, just like your exhaling breath. Hear the water receding in the sound of air exiting your lungs.

8. Continue to "breathe the ocean" in this way. Try to sustain your awareness so the imagined scene effortlessly repeats in sync with your breath cycle.

I AM FILLED WITH LOVING-KINDNESS.

LETTING GO OF EFFORT

PLAYER: 1 | **TIME:** 5 MINUTES

Sometimes life feels hard. We run into a big problem, or many little problems pile up. We try to solve problems using our minds. We review the same information over and over in our head, play out scenarios, and look for ways to get unstuck. When that doesn't work, we criticize ourselves for not being able to find a solution. So we try harder, creating even more stress. But instead of trying so hard to fix what's wrong, what if we asked, "What would make this easier?" In this exercise, you'll use your breath to pause during stressful moments and release the need to fix everything.

---

1. Relax into a comfortable seated position with your eyes closed.

2. Turn your awareness to your breath. Inhale and exhale a few times.

3. Now ask yourself, "Am I watching the breath or controlling the breath?" Consider this question as you let your breath move in and out a few times.

4. Next, start to control your breath. Consciously decide when to inhale and exhale. Exaggerate a little so you feel the experience of controlling the breath. How can you tell that your breath is being controlled? What is your mind doing? What is your body doing? How does it feel?

5. Return to normal breathing. Now simply watch your breath without controlling it. You can be confident that the breath will happen on its own because it's an automatic function of the body. Keep your awareness on simply watching the breath.

6. What is different compared to when you controlled the breath? Notice that your mind is more open when it's not directing action. Feel what it's like to trust your body to breathe on its own.

7. Consider what you need to let go of to simply watch the breath. What else can you do to stop controlling it? You may experience relief from the burden of trying to take control.

8. As you go through your day, see what happens when you bring this steady awareness to life situations that you try to control. Consider what it would look like to let the situations unfold with less effort.

I AM SAFE AND PROTECTED.

DRAWING FROM YOUR INNER WELL

PLAYER: 1 | **TIME:** 5 MINUTES

Innovative psychotherapist Richard Schwartz teaches that all people have inherent positive qualities like calm, clarity, compassion, curiosity, confidence, courage, creativity, and connectedness. With mindfulness, we can bring these traits to the forefront. Use this visualization to help draw forth your positive qualities when you need them, like water from a well.

---

1. Sit in a comfortable upright position. Place your feet securely on the floor. Relax but remain alert.

2. Imagine a water well in your mind's eye. It's a few feet high, lined with stones, and covered by a small roof. Across the opening is a crank wrapped with a rope and a bucket on the end.

3. On the next inhalation, imagine a tiny bucket lowering into your air passage with your breath. Imagine it going down through your nose and into your neck and chest.

4. At the end of your inhalation, notice where the bucket stops. Imagine it coming back to the surface as you exhale.

5. Repeat, allowing your breath to become more relaxed with each cycle. Imagine the bucket gradually reaching the bottom of your lungs, diaphragm, and into your belly.

6. Now imagine a cool, clean natural spring at the bottom of your well. This represents the essence of confidence—secure, stable, and reassuring.

7. On your next inhalation, imagine the bucket filling with a deep sense of confidence from the spring and bringing it up where you can access it. Continue breathing this way until you can sustain a feeling of reassuring security that comes from deep within yourself.

8. Now repeat the steps, but imagine the spring represents caring qualities—feeling loved and respected. Once again, imagine the bucket accessing this loving acceptance from within yourself. Keep breathing until you can sustain this feeling.

9. You can repeat this process with any quality, such as creativity, compassion, and clarity. Trust that each is a resource you can access from deep within yourself.

I AM HEALTHY IN MIND AND BODY.

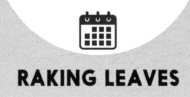

RAKING LEAVES

PLAYER: 1 | **TIME:** VARIABLE

We tend to resist our chores and try to finish them in a hurry so that we can get to the "fun" stuff. As teacher Thich Nhat Hanh wrote in *Peace Is Every Step*, "If I hurry in order to eat dessert sooner, the time of washing dishes will be unpleasant and not worth living. That would be a pity." Tedious tasks are great opportunities to practice mindful awareness. When we are present during such tasks—instead of yearning to be somewhere else—we can improve the quality of our life in those moments. In this activity, you'll practice doing a chore mindfully. I've used raking leaves as an example, but you can adapt this for doing dishes, making the bed, or even working online.

---

1. Prepare to rake leaves. Approach your rake like a fine tool. Respectfully remove it from its resting place, being careful not to disturb other tools. Feel its weight in your hands. Notice its simple, functional design. Appreciate the weathered handle.

2. As you perform the task, sync your breath to the raking motion. Inhale when reaching the rake outward and exhale when pulling it toward you. Use a slow, mindful motion. If you'd like to go faster, breathe in during every two to three raking motions, and then breathe out for two to three raking motions. Try it both fast and slow.

3. Allow each breath to draw your awareness more deeply into the task. Notice when and where your body aches and what the aching feels like. Also notice when your body feels energized. Watch how various physical sensations dissipate and emerge while you're doing the task.

4. If your mind wanders, let the breath be like a tap on the shoulder, reminding you to bring your awareness back to the present moment.

5. When you're ready, pause for a break. Stop all movement and bring awareness to the sensations pulsing through your body. Where is energy flowing the strongest through you?

6. Make note of your progress. Appreciate how your simple, repeating actions gradually reshape your surroundings.

I LIVE WITH EASE AND JOY.

TUNING IN TO RELIEF

We might imagine that mindfulness is all about bliss, peace, and harmony. Photos of people meditating usually shows them with calm, happy faces. No one ever seems to have a toothache or stinging back pain! But, in the real world, physical discomfort and pain happen. Mindfulness shows us that we can experience relief from pain by turning toward it rather than fighting against it. This activity teaches you to use mindfulness as a balm for pain. Note that this practice is meant for manageable aches. If you're in extreme pain or discomfort, seek medical attention.

---

1. Find a comfortable seated position or lie on your back. Try to be both physically relaxed and mentally alert.

2. Once you're comfortable, scan your body. Start at the top of your head, letting your awareness slowly drift downward. Let your awareness glide along your body, inch by inch, all the way down to your feet. Maintain a steady, smooth breath. It's like you're standing in a refreshing stream, washing awareness over yourself.

3. Once you've reached your feet, start over at the top of your head. This time, scan for aches in your body as you go. You may notice many types of sensations—for example, dull pressure in the knees, a kink in the neck, or a knot in the back. Just note them and allow your awareness to keep moving along your body as you breathe.

4. When you're ready, find an ache to focus on and keep your awareness on it. Imagine breathing directly into that location, steadily and slowly, over and over again.

5. As you breathe, consider these questions: What shape is the pain? Where is its boundary? How would you describe it (temperature, sensation, depth)?

6. Observe the pain while you breathe into it for several breaths. Notice the shape, intensity, and quality of the ache change as you breathe into it.

7. Exploring pain in this way can cause it to dissipate or even completely subside. What is your experience?

I CONNECT WITH MY TRUE NATURE.

GIFTS AND GRATITUDE

PLAYERS: 2 OR MORE | **TIME:** 10 TO 15 MINUTES

Gratitude is a simple and powerful tool. When you're feeling blue, remembering what you are grateful for is a reliable and inexpensive way to improve your mood, increase optimism, and deepen relationships. But you don't have to feel down to gain these benefits. Gratitude is closely linked to mindfulness. When we are mindful, we can more easily notice the simple, pervasive beauty of life. And when we see more clearly, it becomes that much easier to appreciate what we already have. In this activity, you'll use the natural breath cycle to practice mindfully expressing gratitude with others to gain the positive benefits of connection.

---

1. Sit comfortably across from each other or in a circle.

2. Players begin by paying attention to their breath and centering themselves with a few deep breaths.

3. Together, take a deep inhalation and long, slow exhalation.

4. Each person takes a turn saying, "Inhaling, I appreciate the gift of *(fill in the blank)*. Exhaling, I give thanks to/for *(fill in the blank)*." If you wish, players can take several turns.

▶ **TIP:** The "gifts and gratitude" statement can be adapted to many situations. For example, each player can name specific qualities they appreciate about another player to foster group cohesion. Or players can name a firsthand experience during inhalation, and then give thanks to something they observed between others during exhalation. Moreover, if you are going through a hardship, this activity can help the group discover positive lessons from within a difficult situation.

I AM THE STEWARD OF MY MIND.

TAPPING INTO YOUR INNER MUSICIAN

PLAYERS: 2 OR MORE | **TIME:** 5 MINUTES

Evidence suggests that making music may have been important to human evolution. In fact, we may have been singers before we were speakers! Unfortunately, most of us don't make music and concede that pleasure to those with "talent." We may sing in the shower but become embarrassed around others. This is too bad, since singing has traditionally been an important part of building community. Mindfulness helps us reconnect with our basic ability to make music. In this activity, you'll use the breath to create melodic sounds and build community.

---

1. Sit comfortably across from each other or in a circle. Briefly describe the sound that is made by moving air through our vocal cords. When we talk, we quickly piece together these sounds into words and sentences. By making just one sound at a time and holding it, we can discover that the body is naturally built to make music.

2. One player volunteers to make a roller-coaster "melody" by gently holding a long "o" sound at a comfortable pitch in the middle of their vocal range. As the player holds the sound, they gradually slide lower and higher in their range. (Singers should stay where most people can access the range without difficulty.)

3. Now the other players join by following the first player's lead on when to raise and lower the range. Each player should stay with whatever pitch feels best to them. Notice that, as everyone

sustains their sounds, there is a tendency to sync into simple harmonization, like a choir!

4. The lead player now introduces a mindful breath by saying, "Inhale, 1...2...3...4..." while the others inhale. Then everyone exhales while making the long "o" roller-coaster melody. Repeat this step two to four times to further sync the group and bring awareness to the breath's important role in singing.

5. You can repeat with different players taking the lead for another round or next time.

➧ **TIP:** There are many variations of this activity. For example, try using different vowels, impersonate whale song, or pretend to have a conversation with just one sustained vowel.

I RELAX AND DO MY BEST; THE UNIVERSE DOES THE REST.

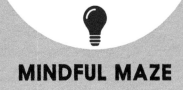

MINDFUL MAZE

People around the world have built mazes since ancient times. Walking through these mazes cultivated contemplation and mindful awareness. The maze is a metaphor for life. There are long and short paths, meandering turns, and a sense of ongoing discovery. In a maze, we practice valuing each step, rather than focusing on "getting somewhere." Use the maze on the next page to practice mindful breathing. Simply trace the maze with your finger.

---

1. Find a table or a surface where the maze can lie flat.

2. Sit up straight, relax your jaw and shoulders, and place your feet securely on the floor. Calmly breathe in and out three to four times to center yourself.

3. Begin drawing a path through the maze in sync with your breath. Inhale to the count of four as you proceed to the first turn. Move your finger slowly enough so it reaches the next turn at the top of your inhalation.

4. Exhale to the count of four as you turn and proceed down the next section of path. Time your exhalation so it completes just as you arrive at the next turn.

5. Continue inhaling and exhaling between turns. On longer stretches between turns, you'll notice that you move your finger more quickly to sync it with your breathing.

6. Observe the tendency of your mind to react in different ways: impatient, relaxed, bored, calm. Return awareness to the breath and your finger on the page when your mind tries to intervene.

7. Explore the entire maze, and finish when you reach "end." What connections do you see between the experience of tracing the labyrinth and the path you're walking in life?

➡ **TIP:** Some days, you may want to complete the labyrinth as quickly as possible. Other days, you may want to retrace sections to extend the practice.

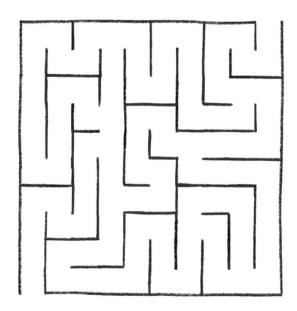

THE WELLNESS WHEEL

PLAYER: 1 | **TIME:** 5 TO 10 MINUTES | **SUPPLIES:** COLORED PENCILS

The imagination is a powerful force. Athletes, actors, chess champions, and tech tycoons have all used visualization to help make their dreams come true. There's evidence that visualization has both psychological (improved confidence) and physical (improved strength) benefits. We can use visualization in our personal lives, too. This exercise combines breath, drawing, and visualization to help you create a vision of your future self in various aspects of life. May your vision of wellness become reality!

---

1. Choose four wellness categories for your Wellness Wheel, such as purpose, personal growth, friends/family, romantic relationship(s), mental health, physical health, and fun/recreation.

2. Write one category on the line beside each of the four sections of the Wellness Wheel on the next page.

3. Pick one category and choose a color. Doodle in the wheel slice for that category. As you doodle, reflect on your vision for that area of life. For example, "Regarding my life purpose, I see myself becoming *(fill in the blank)*." Doodle slowly, syncing your breath with the movement of your hand. You can make any type of doodle, such as squiggles, repeating shapes, and figures.

4. Switch colors. Now doodle in another category. Continue to sync the breath with the movement of your hand and reflect on your vision for that category. For example, "Regarding my friends and family, I see myself becoming *(fill in the blank)*."

5. Repeat for the remaining categories with different colors.

6. The finished Wellness Wheel represents your future vision. Take a few minutes to scan the doodles and recall the different aspects of your vision. Then close your eyes and imagine how you would feel if these visions became reality. As you breathe in, let the delight of your vision follow your breath and fill your body all the way down to your toes. As you exhale, imagine offering the world your vision as a gift.

➡ **TIP:** Over time, you'll likely notice your future vision changes, and that is okay! The doodles playfully represent the spontaneous, flowing rhythm of life's unpredictable twists and turns.

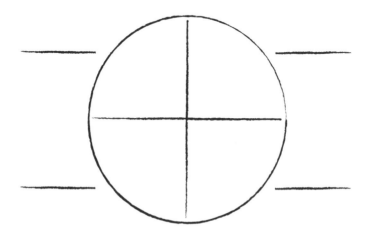

MIND

2

THE ORBIT OF AWARENESS

PLAYER: 1 | **TIME:** 5 MINUTES

Do you know where your awareness is located? Most of us experience awareness as being just behind our eyes. We might think of consciousness as being in our brain and that our awareness looks out from the eyes. It can seem that awareness and thoughts are the same thing. Actually, we can move our awareness with great agility. In this activity, you'll practice moving your awareness, which can help you see that you are more than your thoughts.

---

1. Sit comfortably and close your eyes. Place your feet securely on the floor, sit up a little straighter, and take a few calming breaths.

2. Once you're settled, bring your awareness to the space behind your head, just above your neck. This will be similar to feeling the presence of someone behind you. Simply tune your awareness in to that "what's behind you" type of knowing.

3. Now gently and slowly move your awareness forward along both sides of your head.

4. Continue moving your awareness forward along both sides until you reach the edges of your peripheral vision. It will be approximately just behind your temples.

5. Keep your awareness there for a moment. Observe the unique experience of being aware of what's just beyond the edge of your field of vision.

6. When you're ready, continue to move your awareness forward around both sides of your head. Continue until the awareness coming from the left meets the awareness coming from the right in front of your head. As awareness meets awareness, you realize you've been holding awareness in two locations at once. Kind of weird. Kind of cool!

7. Finally, hold the full orbit you just completed in your awareness. Be aware of the entire ring of space around your head at once. Relax into this full-orbit awareness for as long as you like.

8. Congrats! You moved awareness outside of your thinking mind. Where else might you take it?

I CHOOSE AND CREATE MY INNER EXPERIENCE.

WELCOME, MONKEYS!

PLAYER: 1 | **TIME:** 10 MINUTES

Have you ever felt your mind in overdrive? Thoughts race from one topic to the next, chaotic and in a never-ending loop. Buddhism refers to this as "monkey mind." It's hard to see life clearly with a monkey mind. Things appear fast and furious, so we grasp tightly to get control. But in reality, it's our perception causing the chaos. Somewhere inside we know this, and it makes us critical toward our monkey mind. Instead of criticizing, it works better to befriend the monkeys. How? Get to know them! This simple exercise helps tame the monkey mind.

---

1. Prepare to interview your monkey mind. This isn't a job interview; it's more like getting to know someone. You are both the interviewer and the monkey, asking questions to gain understanding and appreciation. Have fun with this: Use different voices, move between chairs, or wear different hats in each role.

2. Before asking questions, pause. You might say, "Monkey mind, can we take a moment to get settled? Let's sit up straighter, put our feet firmly on the ground, and take two slow breaths." Then ask the questions, listen for the responses, and respond to them, as follows:

   ➧ "Thank you for letting me get to know you better. I notice you are acting frantically. I care for your well-being. Could you share what worries you?"

- "That's understandable. What is your job in responding to this situation? What do you feel is your responsibility?"

- "What are you afraid will happen if you don't do your job?"

- "What is your positive intention? What do you want for me?"

- After you've explored these questions, say, "Thank you so much for trying to help me in this way." Then recall times in life when the monkey has played this role and it's helped you. Express acknowledgment and appreciation for the monkey's efforts.

- Finally, say, "I really appreciate your help. How might we address this situation in a way that you can remain calm and relaxed?"

3. Brainstorm options with your monkey mind and then try one out!

I LISTEN TO THE CALL THAT LONGS TO LIVE THROUGH ME.

FILL THE MIND WITH NATURE

PLAYER: 1 | **TIME:** 10 MINUTES

Sometimes the mind fills itself up with all the distractions going on around us. Whomever or whatever we give our awareness to will become the focus of our thoughts, emotions, and actions. When we give the gift of our awareness away, it gradually becomes more difficult to fend off nagging distractions. This activity exercises your ability to choose where your awareness goes. A setting in nature, free from electronics, screens, and other demands for your attention, can teach you how to choose the content of your mind.

1. Find a comfortable place to sit outside such as a park, wooded area, beach, or even your yard or patio.

2. Sit straight and relaxed, as though there's a string gently holding you upright from the top of your head. Take a full, relaxing breath. Feel the weight of your body as an organism on the Earth.

3. Now close your eyes and turn your awareness to sound. Allow the content of your mind to become only the sounds you hear. Imagine the sounds as thoughts moving through your mind. Continue this for one to two minutes.

4. Next, open your eyes and turn your awareness to what you are seeing. Look around at the shapes and shadows of the environment you're in. Soften your eyes to see your entire field of vision at once. Let the images you see replace the thoughts in your mind.

Continue this for one to two minutes. Let the items in the environment become the content of your mind.

5. Close your eyes and turn your awareness to touch. Let the sensations of wind, clothing, what you are sitting on, and what your hands are resting on become the content of your mind. Sustain awareness of touch for one to two minutes.

6. Finally, open your eyes and tune in to all three senses at once: sound, sight, and touch. How does it feel to fill your mind this way? How might choosing where your awareness goes help you be more mindful in your daily life?

I REMAIN OPENHEARTED EVEN WHEN I FEEL STRESSED.

KNOWING BEYOND THINKING

PLAYER: 1 | **TIME:** 5 MINUTES

In Western traditions, the thinking brain is given privileged status as the location where information is stored and processed. Many Eastern mindfulness traditions teach that the mind is just one of many organs that contribute to insight. For example, studies show that the heart and gut also have neurons like the brain. When we focus only on logic and ideas, we may miss important information that the brain can't access alone. Integrating head, heart, and gut provides insight that can lead to better decisions. Use this meditation to help you access other innate sources of intelligence beyond thoughts.

---

1. Sit in a comfortable position and prepare to turn inward by taking a few breaths. Close your eyes, sit up straight, and place your feet securely on the floor.

2. Bring awareness to the space around your eyes. Typically, we experience the location of our consciousness in our head, looking out at the world from our eyes. Tune in to that feeling. Notice if there is any tightness in the muscles around your eyes. If so, gently allow it to release.

3. Slowly move awareness below your eyes to the areas around the cheekbones and jaw. Again, notice any tightness and gently allow it to release.

4. Next, let your awareness move into your throat. Notice the sensations of the throat, around the airways and within the vocal cords. Simply tune in to the sense of throat awareness.

5. Now drop your awareness into the area of your heart. Sense your lungs expanding and contracting as you breathe. Be aware of how the rib cage gently holds space for the movement of your breath. Imagine breathing directly into the wide expanse of your loving heart.

6. Maintaining awareness in your heart, note how your gut, heart, and brain exchange information. Outside your body, information arrives in the form of smells, conversations, and news. It mingles with information from inside you, like tingling sensations, thoughts, and hopes. Appreciate that you are complex, integrated, and whole.

7. Ask yourself, "What really matters at this point in my life? What issues would like more attention? What is my greatest source of internal happiness?" Quietly listen to the wisdom of your mind-heart-gut brain.

I AM CREATIVE, RESOURCEFUL, AND WHOLE.

FROM DOING TO BEING

PLAYER: 1 | **TIME:** 5 MINUTES

We live in the age of doing. We keep full schedules, organize massive to-do lists, and strategize better ways of getting things done. Being busy seems to indicate we're on the right track. But all this doing can cause harm. We can use it to avoid our feelings. We can fill life with activity rather than the relationships and reflection that give life meaning. Inspired by meditation teacher Loch Kelly's practice "No Problem to Solve," this exercise will help you experience being human rather than doing human.

---

1. Sit upright in a comfortable, alert position and take a few breaths to center yourself. Keep your eyes open.

2. Tune in to the sense of yourself as a "doer" whose consciousness is right behind your eyes. Look around the room and notice what is out of place that the mind wants to fix.

3. Notice what else your mind wants to do—for example, make a list, comment on this experience, or look at your phone. Notice how it wants to grab at and fidget with all kinds of mental tasks.

4. Take a full inhalation and slowly exhale. Now simply notice what remains when you stop trying to do anything with your mind. Observe for several moments. When you stop doing, you don't stop existing. Observe what's left of your existence.

5. When your body is still, you get a different experience of being in your body. You might become more attuned to sensations like pulsing, throbbing, and temperature. The same is true when your mind is still. It shifts from the narrowness of thinking to the expansiveness of awareness. You become attuned to the simple, direct experience of being aware.

6. Notice what comes to your awareness. What is left of who you are? What qualities come to the forefront?

GRATITUDE TRANSFORMS AN ANXIOUS MIND.

MINDFUL LISTENING

PLAYER: 1 | **TIME:** 5 MINUTES

There's an interesting difference between how we access sights and sounds. When we direct our gaze on an object, it's like we "grab" it with our sight. But we hear sounds more holistically, receiving whatever sound waves flow toward us. In this way, hearing is a less active and more accepting sense than seeing. Tuning in to your sense of hearing can be a relaxing way to practice being receptive, even in busy times. Enjoy how this short listening activity creates a feeling of spacious calm.

1. Lie comfortably on a couch, bed, or floor. Use pillows or other props to caringly nestle yourself into a position that feels relieving. Get as comfortable as you can.

2. Take four breaths that gradually grow longer and deeper. Feel the pressure of the surface you're lying on.

3. Close your eyes and tune in to your sense of hearing. Try to sustain your awareness on nothing but the sounds you hear.

4. Notice sounds in your room, such as a furnace or air conditioner, the creaking of walls, and the buzzing of appliances. Include sounds you make when gently repositioning yourself and sounds that come from within you: your breathing, heartbeat, or gurgling in your belly.

5. Shift your awareness to sounds outside, such as birds, wind, raindrops, or cars passing by.

6. Tune in to the farthest away sound you can hear.

7. Tune in to the sound that originates closest to your ears.

8. Imagine all the sounds you are hearing traveling through a huge, spacious sky. As you listen, imagine their sound waves rippling through the air.

9. When thoughts arise, imagine the words that make up those thoughts floating across the sky alongside the sound waves. Watch them pass by and out of sight like clouds.

10. When you're ready, open your eyes and take a deep breath. Consider what seems most important from this place of calm awareness.

THE UNIVERSE HAS UNFOLDED TO INCLUDE ME.

CLEARING OUT MENTAL CHATTER

PLAYERS: 2 | **TIME:** 45 MINUTES | **SUPPLIES:** TIMER

We spend most of our time in our heads. And who can blame us? So many attention-grabbing things happen there. Dreams and fantasies! Worries, doubts, and criticisms! Things we should have said! All this mental activity brings challenges. It's nearly impossible to communicate it all. It can distract us from seeing situations clearly. Worst of all, thoughts, worries, etc. can make us feel stuck, anxious, and overwhelmed. What if we could dump thoughts like taking out the trash? In this exercise, each player takes turns verbalizing their thoughts to clear out mental "noise" and gain a clearer perspective.

---

1. Find a safe, private place to have a one-on-one conversation where both players feel at ease.

2. Get comfortable and face each other. Decide who will be player 1 and who will be player 2.

3. Set the timer for 10 minutes. Player 1 says whatever comes into their mind, letting the thoughts pour out in a stream of consciousness, speaking constantly. Player 2 remains silent and attentive. No interruptions.

4. When the timer goes off, switch roles and repeat step 3. The idea is for player 2 to let their own thoughts pour out rather than use their time to respond to player 1's thoughts.

5. Now set the timer for five minutes. Repeat step 3, and then reset the timer and switch places to repeat step 3 one more time.

6. Set the timer for three minutes and sit together in silence, placing your gaze wherever feels comfortable.

7. When the timer goes off, compare notes on how it felt to share. Try not to focus on the content that was shared. Instead, talk about the range of feelings that surfaced both when you were the listener and when you were the speaker. Were there any surprises? Do you feel inspired to take any action now that you've cleared out the mental clutter?

RIGHT. NOW. IS. JUST. THIS.

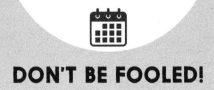

DON'T BE FOOLED!

PLAYERS: 3 TO 5 | **TIME:** 30 MINUTES PER PLAYER

Sometimes we fool ourselves in an effort to fool someone else. Why would we do this? Perhaps we don't want to feel vulnerable, so we tell ourselves we don't care about a criticism. Or we don't want to hurt a romantic partner by breaking up with them, so we convince ourselves we're in love. When we fool ourselves, we're often the last to know! We lose touch with our truth and can't see all our choices. This activity can help you open up new possibilities by seeing your situation through the eyes of others. Taking turns exploring situations in one another's lives can be a fun and meaningful way to spend an evening with close friends.

---

1. Identify a situation in life where you can't move forward, keep repeating a similar mistake, or are unsure of what to do next.

2. Summarize the situation in three to five minutes, making sure to include who, what, when, where, why, and how. Then, ask, "How might I be fooling myself in this situation?"

3. All the other players take a turn coming up with possible alternatives to the who, what, when, where, why, and how. The goal is to offer plausible alternatives that explain the situation in a new way. Players should not try to solve each other's problem, just offer a fresh perspective.

4. Once everyone has offered a possible alternative, discuss any emerging insights into your situation. Did you hear anything unexpected? Can you use this expanded awareness to create a new way forward?

5. Repeat steps 1 to 4 for each player, so that everyone has a chance to share and reflect.

➡ **TIP:** You can do this activity as a group or with each person individually.

RELAXING, I LET MYSELF SIMPLY BE.

HACKING YOUR OWN CODE

PLAYER: 1 | **TIME:** 5 TO 10 MINUTES
SUPPLIES: JOURNAL AND PEN OR VIRTUAL NOTEPAD

Computers get updated all the time. Some updates are major overhauls; others make minor tweaks. By changing computer code, developers can fix bugs so that their programs work as well as possible. In life, we can also develop "bugs" in our system. These bugs include beliefs about ourselves that can limit our happiness, joy, and overall well-being. With awareness, we can learn to change these beliefs! This exercise explores how you might begin changing limiting beliefs by mindfully adopting new ones.

---

1. Look over the list of beliefs on the next page. If you could "download" one and believe it wholeheartedly, resulting in a significant upgrade in your life, which would it be?

2. Scan your memory and identify a time when you acted on that belief. Like replaying a video, notice what you were doing, how you felt, and what the circumstances were that allowed you to live in alignment with this belief.

3. Now, identify a present-day problem that could improve if you had this belief in your current operating system. What strategies have you tried to address the problem? Have you tried those strategies before? Be compassionate with yourself here, knowing that all our behaviors—even undesirable coping mechanisms—are well-intentioned attempts to serve us in some way.

4. Now, imagine that you have downloaded this belief into your mind and that it overwrites any conflicting beliefs. How might you address your current problem with this new programming?

5. In your journal or notepad, brainstorm a list of actions that might flow from this wholehearted belief. Which of these actions do you feel most ready to take?

List of Beliefs

I am enough.	I'm doing my best.	I am safe.	Both perspectives can be true.
I can move forward even when it's hard.	I will keep trying.	I can learn to do this.	There's more than one way to get things done.
I approve of myself.	I am creative and resourceful.	I don't need to be in control.	I can learn from others.
I can make room for others when I'm under stress.	Everyone's perspective matters.	I can forgive others.	I am whole.

I ACCEPT MY FULL SELF.

THE MIND IN THE WILD

PLAYER: 1 | **TIME:** 5 MINUTES OR LESS, AT THE TOP OF EACH WAKING HOUR | **SUPPLIES:** PEN AND PAPER OR VIRTUAL NOTEPAD AND A TIMER

A mindfulness practice is like watching birds at a bird feeder. If we watch casually, we see a random assortment of birds coming and going. But if we observe closely, patterns emerge. Different species tend to feed at certain times of day. We notice the same individual birds again and again because their nest is nearby. Others stop just once on the way to someplace else. In this activity, you'll observe your mind's patterns "in the wild," similar to keeping field notes as birds come and go from the feeder. This activity helps you start becoming more aware of what's going on in your mind.

---

1. Set your timer to go off at the top of each waking hour.

2. Create a simple three-column table on paper or a virtual notepad. Label column 1 "time," column 2 "thought," and column 3 "positive/negative/neutral."

3. When the timer goes off, tune in to your thoughts. Simply observe them like they are visiting birds. Pull out your chart and jot down the time in column 1, the thought(s) in column 2, and note if the thought(s) have a positive, negative, or neutral tone in column 3.

4. Review your field notes at the end of the day. Which "birds" visited your "feeder" and when? How many different varieties (topics) showed up? Was there a dominant tone of positive, negative, or neutral? Did any thoughts lessen in importance as the day wore on? What insight have you gained from mindfully observing the feeder of your mind? Can you put out seeds to attract the more positive birds in the future?

▶ **TIP:** You can invite someone you know to keep a field record, too, and compare your notes at the end of the day. If you like this activity, try it for a week or longer. You may want to keep separate field notes for work and home, or weekdays and weekend. Notice how the patterns change in these different contexts.

I PRACTICE GRATITUDE AND NOURISH MY BODY AND MIND.

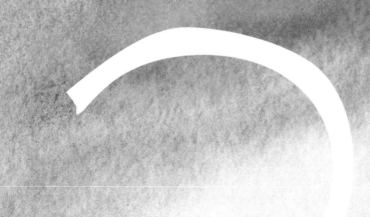

BODY

SENSORY IMMERSION TANK

PLAYER: 1 | **TIME:** 10 MINUTES
SUPPLIES: OPTIONAL YOGA MAT, PILLOWS, CANDLES

A sensory deprivation tank is a dark, soundproof tank filled with body-temperature salt water in which a person floats and experiences virtually no external stimuli. This is done for therapeutic benefits, such as pain relief and reduced anxiety. Of course, sensory deprivation tanks aren't available to everyone. What's ironic is that we can gain similar benefits by doing the exact opposite! In this activity, you'll immerse yourself in an imaginary *sensory immersion* tank to generate heightened, mindful awareness of your senses. Linger as long as you like on any sense.

---

1. Go to a location where you can practice uninterrupted awareness for at least 10 minutes. Complete silence isn't necessary.

2. Build your tank (i.e., a comfortable place to lie down). You could arrange pillows on your favorite couch, prepare a cozy bed, place candles around a yoga mat, or find a peaceful nook in nature.

3. Enter the tank by slowly easing yourself into a reclined position. Imagine slipping into a gentle, nourishing bath. You can keep your eyes open or closed.

4. Once settled, bring your awareness to the sensation of touch in your feet. Slowly move awareness from your feet up along your body, focusing on the sense of touch. Notice any warm, tingling sensation that signals aliveness in your body. Notice temperature, texture, and softness. Guide your awareness all the way to the top of your head.

5. Now bring your awareness to sound. What sounds are farthest away? Which are nearby? Which are coming from you? Experiment with simply hearing instead of listening. Rather than trying to identify the sounds, simply hear them arise and subside.

6. Shift your awareness to your sense of smell. Breathe in the air and immerse yourself in the sensation of smelling.

7. Shift your awareness to your sense of taste. Notice tastes present in your mouth without identifying what they are.

8. Open your eyes (if closed) and bring your awareness to what you see. There's no need to move your head and look around. Simply see what is in front of you.

9. Stay present in the relaxing sensory experiences happening right now for as long as you'd like.

I LISTEN MINDFULLY TO OTHERS.

BUILD A BODY DASHBOARD

PLAYER: 1 | **TIME:** 10 TO 15 MINUTES
SUPPLIES: PAPER AND COLORED PENCILS, MARKERS, OR CRAYONS

The dashboard of a car tracks speed, engine temperature, fuel level, and more to help us operate the vehicle. Our bodies provide information that helps us operate, too. Most of us are good at reading our bodies' physical signals, like sleepiness or hunger, but we often miss the emotional information that accompanies physical cues. Being mindful of the subtle links between emotions and physical sensations can help us understand ourselves better, communicate more clearly, and skillfully respond, rather than overreact, to our experiences. In this exercise, you'll build a dashboard to track your body's emotional signals and get to know them better.

---

1. Make three equal columns on a piece of paper in landscape orientation. Label the left column "physical sensations," and label the right column "emotions."

2. In the middle column, draw a body. It can be detailed, cartoonish, or simply a stick figure. Include the whole body from head to feet.

3. In the left column, list as many physical sensations as you can think of: tingling, pulsing, cool, tight, etc. Leave room to add others as you experience them.

4. In the right column, list as many emotions as you can think of: happy, sad, excited, nervous, anxious, bored, etc. Again, leave some room to add others.

5. You've just created your body dashboard! Now, give it a test run. Identify the emotion you're feeling right now. Find it on the list or add it if needed. Circle the emotion in a color you associate with the emotion (for example, red for angry and blue for sad).

6. Now turn your awareness to your body. What physical sensations indicate that you are feeling that emotion? Look closely. Using the same color, underline the physical sensation(s) in the first column. (Write it in first if it's not already listed.) Mark an *X* on the body in the middle column where you feel that sensation.

7. You can keep your dashboard handy throughout the day to identify the links between your physical sensations and emotions.

I CHOOSE WHAT TO DO WITH MY TIME.

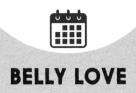

BELLY LOVE

PLAYER: 1 | **TIME:** 10 MINUTES

Take a moment to consider what the belly does for us. It digests food and creates energy, and we rely on its "gut instincts" to make important choices. But we rarely offer back the care and attention our bellies deserve. In fact, the belly is often where stress accumulates. Stress can lead to uncomfortable stomach sensations like tightness, twisting, and nausea. Meditation teacher Roshi Joan Halifax teaches the importance of having a strong back and a soft belly: A wholehearted life requires both inner confidence (a strong back) and vulnerability (a soft belly). This activity gives you a chance to relax your belly and mindfully nurture your ability to meet the world with love and openness.

---

1. Lie comfortably on your back or side. Close your eyes. Visualize any tension dissolving into the surface beneath you.

2. Place your hands tenderly on your belly, as though resting your hand on an infant or pet. Feel the rise and fall of your belly as you breathe.

3. Shift awareness to the space within your belly. Note what you sense there. For example, there may be tightness, gurgling, pressure, or a simple sense of space.

4. Check for any remaining tightness. Take a deep breath, then push all the air out. Allow your belly to be completely loose and supple, with nothing but gravity holding it.

5. Connect with the internal associations you have with your belly. What memories come to the surface? What emotions are linked with it? What does your belly remind you of?

6. Notice whether the associations have positive, negative, or neutral undertones. When you notice a negative connotation, offer your belly acknowledgment and appreciation. For example, you might say, "I see you are burdened with criticism for being flabby. I appreciate that you hold my stress when I don't know where else to put it."

7. Rub your hands over your belly compassionately. Allow yourself to feel tenderly comforted by your own loving touch.

8. Finally, imagine your belly as a source of openhearted energy. What does it feel like to let your belly be open and loving? How can you express this energy in daily life?

I SPEAK TO BE UNDERSTOOD.

INTUITION CHECK-IN

PLAYER: 1 | **TIME:** 5 TO 10 MINUTES (PLUS TIME FOR ACTIVITIES)

When we're in a "flow state," time flies by, but we don't feel rushed. We are productive without becoming exhausted. Whether cooking dinner or doing a more complex task, life feels great when we're in the flow. Unfortunately, flow states can be unpredictable and hard to access. So, we use other ways of getting things done, such as planning, setting deadlines, and pushing through distractions. These approaches get the job done but use a lot of energy. With this activity, you can learn to access the flow state more often by mindfully tuning in to your intuition.

1. Prepare or review your day's to-do list.

2. Begin with a brief body-clearing: Stand up and shake your body for 5 to 15 seconds. Wiggle your arms, legs, and torso. Give your head a good shake.

3. Slowly lift your arms windmill-style as you slowly inhale. Touch your hands at the top of your inhalation. Pause, then slowly lower your arms as you exhale. Exaggerate the slowness. You might feel a pulsing sensation as you lower your arms.

4. Now ask your body, "What is the most energizing thing I can do first?" Scan your body for a response. Let an answer emerge without using your logical brain. For instance, your intuition might tell you to meditate or answer a particular email before diving into a big report. Do that.

5. When the activity is complete, choose your next activity the same way. Ask yourself "sensing" questions ("What do I feel most called to do?" "What do I feel ready for now?" and "What can I do joy-fully?") rather than hierarchical questions ("What is most urgent?" "What is most challenging?" and "What do I HAVE to do?")

6. Throughout the day, work on the activities that have the strongest resonance with your intuition. Trust that your instincts are giving you good advice. Notice when you begin to lose focus or energy. Instead of powering through. Ask your body, "What kind of break would be most helpful?" Do that for 5 to 10 minutes.

7. After the break, ask your body, "What's next?" Continue this way, relying on your intuition to guide how you spend your time. At day's end, reflect on how this experience compares to how you normally approach tasks.

I AM WILLING TO CHANGE.

STRETCHING BOUNDARIES

PLAYER: 1 | **TIME:** 5 MINUTES

Have you ever marveled at your ability to sense that someone is behind you? Or that someone is staring at you without looking at them? Or that you can navigate tight spaces like a crowded dance floor without bumping into anyone? We can do these things because human perception is incredibly sophisticated. We can even extend the sense of our physical boundary beyond our bodies to include tools we're using—like when driving a car, using a spatula, or mowing the lawn. In this exercise, you'll explore how to stretch your sense of self beyond your physical body to enhance mindful awareness.

---

1. Sit comfortably in an upright, relaxed position. Place your feet securely on the floor. Rest your hands in front of you on your legs, a pillow on your lap, or a table.

2. Open and close your hands three to five times, stretching your fingers out and then closing them into fists. This will get the blood flowing and increase the sensations in your hands. Place them open with palms down when you're finished.

3. Now close your eyes and bring your awareness to the sensations in your hands. Notice the strongest sensations like pulsing, tingling, or warmth. They may also include the pressure of your hands against the surface they are resting upon.

4. Shift your awareness to the inside of your hands. Consider what's inside your fingers. Turn your awareness to the small, internal spaces between your bones, muscles, and veins. Consider the place where your hands become your wrists.

5. Now bring awareness to the boundary between your hands and the space around them. Mentally outline the edge of your hand. What are you noticing? Where do your hands end and the space around them begin? How would you describe the boundary?

6. Finally, move awareness to the space above the top of your hand. How far above your hand can you connect with a sense of space? Do the same beneath your hand, like a cushion of air that your palm is resting upon. Try to run your awareness along the edge of each finger like tracing your hand on paper: up one side, over the fingertip, and down the other side. How far can you stretch your awareness beyond the physical boundary of your hand?

I AM ALREADY SAFE.

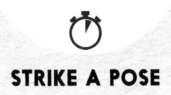

STRIKE A POSE

PLAYER: 1 | **TIME:** 5 MINUTES

Did you know you can use body language to change your mood and behavior? Studies have shown that simply arranging the body into certain poses can create feelings that are consistent with those postures. For example, striking high-power poses can lower stress hormones and increase confidence. Use this technique to put yourself into a more positive mindset when you're feeling down or need a pick-me-up. This works best when you are dealing with negative emotions.

---

1. Stand up and bring your awareness to how you feel. Use two to three adjectives to describe how you're feeling right now, like *worried, doubtful, irritated,* or *uncomfortable.*

2. Spread your legs shoulder-width apart. Lift your chest and head and put your hands on your hips with your elbows pointed out. Bring a look of self-assurance and possibility to your face. This is the Superman pose. Hold this pose for a few breaths and notice any changes in your emotions. How do you feel different?

3. With your legs in the same position, stretch your arms upward at 45-degree angles. Spread out your fingers and take up as much space as you can. Make a facial expression full of brightness. This is the star pose. Hold this pose for a few breaths. How do you feel now?

➧ **TIP:** Find a private spot and try these poses when you are feeling nervous, like before an interview or an important conversation, or anytime you need a confidence boost.

I AM CURIOUS AND COMPASSIONATE WHEN I FEEL RESISTANCE.

FEEL THE RHYTHM

PLAYERS: 4 TO 10 | **TIME:** 15 MINUTES

We all have a natural rhythm that paces our movement. This rhythm is linked to our heart rate, which acts like a hidden, personalized metronome. When our natural rhythm interacts with other people's natural rhythms, unique group dynamics emerge. This team building activity helps players learn to be more mindful of their unique place as part of a team. It also helps team members appreciate the energy and creativity that emerge when they work together.

---

1. Go to an open space, preferably outdoors. A playground or ball field works great.

2. All players stand in a line along one side of the open space. Everyone locates their pulse by placing their index and middle finger alongside their necks.

3. Once the pulse is located, players tap their feet in sync with their heartbeat (their base rhythm).

4. One player says "Go," and all players walk across the open space in sync with their base rhythm, one step per heartbeat.

5. When all players have reached the other side, discuss what each of you noticed about the walk.

6. Repeat steps 2 and 3, but now everyone taps one hand against their leg at a different pace that complements their foot-tapping. This creates a more complex rhythm (and maybe some giggling).

7. Again, one player says "Go," and all players walk across the open space in sync with their more complex rhythm. This time, the "walk" will look more like the ambling procession of a jazz band.

8. When all players have reached the other side, discuss how this walk was different from the first one.

9. Now, everyone lines up again and walks across the space a final time using the complex rhythm, but now they must zigzag into other players' paths and interact with one another, like bees in a beehive. Have fun with this dancing migration across the space!

10. When all players have reached the other side, discuss what each of you noticed about yourself while doing this exercise. When did you feel "in the flow"? When did you feel uncertain? How did other players' movements affect your own? How does this activity mirror the group's interactions in everyday life?

I SPEAK TO MYSELF WITH A CARING HEART.

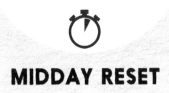

MIDDAY RESET

PLAYERS: 1 OR MORE | **TIME:** 5 MINUTES

Most of us spend a lot of time sitting at a desk, in a car, or on a couch. This isn't what the human body is made for! Studies show that being sedentary has a negative effect on the heart, back, blood circulation, and long-term mental functioning. The good news is that even short physical breaks can have meaningful impacts on health. Combining mindfulness with brief physical activity can provide a nourishing midday reset. Use this short visualization to reboot during long meetings, car trips, or an afternoon of screen time.

1. If you are with other people, propose a short break to stretch. You can invite them to join you or find a private area.

2. Place your feet shoulder-width apart. Slowly windmill your arms up high above your head and then keep them there. Reach to the sky and feel the stretch along both sides of your body.

3. With your arms raised, take a few deep breaths. As you inhale, imagine bringing joyful light into your body. On the exhalation, imagine releasing tiredness, aching, and negativity. With each breath, imagine filling the emptied space with joyful light. Visualize packing it into the microscopic spaces between your cells.

4. Lower your arms on the next exhalation, maintaining awareness of your arms all the way down, until they hang loosely at your sides.

5. Finally, shake your body, section by section. Begin by shaking the left leg, then the right. Then the left and right arm. Shake and twist your torso, and end with a gentle head jiggle. Notice how you feel now and then get back to your day.

I ATTUNE TO THE ALIVENESS PULSING THROUGH ME.

WINDOW OF TOLERANCE

PLAYER: 1 | **TIME:** 5 MINUTES

When we experience stressful situations, the body prepares to fight or flee from the stress. This might cause the heart to beat faster and put us on guard. Or we might shut down, feeling numb or withdrawn. Either way, we lose the ability to think clearly or learn new things, which can lead to poor decisions. But when we practice mindfulness, we can respond another way, remaining calm and relaxed, yet insightful and alert. Use this exercise to practice being in what Daniel Siegel, the executive director of the Mindsight Institute, calls the "window of tolerance." This can help you stay balanced and engaged even in difficult circumstances.

---

1. Take a look at the window of tolerance scale on the next page.

   ◆ **Freeze response (1 to 3).** The physical characteristics of this state include low energy and decreased heart rate. Emotions include feeling withdrawn, numb, and depressed.

   ◆ **Window of tolerance (4 to 7).** In this state, the heart rate is normal and energy is alert and relaxed. Feelings include being calm, curious, and open to any experience.

   ◆ **Fight-or-flight response (8 to 10).** The heart rate is increased and energy is hypervigilant. Feelings include anxiety, reactivity, and defensiveness.

2. Where would you place yourself on the window of tolerance scale in the present moment?

3. Recall times in life when you were far on the "fight-or-flight" end of the spectrum. How about "freeze"? What helped you return to being calm and relaxed in those situations? These examples show that you already have an ability to regulate yourself after stress. Acknowledge this important skill!

4. When you find you're moving out of the window of tolerance, use other activities in this book to recenter yourself. "Breathing the Ocean" on page 4 is a great antidote to fight or flight. "Laughing Meditation" on page 104 works well when we withdraw into freeze.

➡ **TIP:** With practice, you will find that your window of tolerance "opens," meaning you are able to stay calm, alert, and relaxed in a broader range of stressful situations.

	10
Fight or Flight	9
	8
	7
	6
Window of Tolerance	5
	4
	3
Freeze	2
	1

SENSATIONAL WORDS

PLAYER: 1 | **TIME:** 5 MINUTES | **SUPPLIES:** COLORED PENCILS, MARKERS, OR CRAYONS

Have you ever struggled to find the right word? It's an odd feeling, like searching through the brain's closets for a missing shoe. You know it's in here somewhere! Our ability to express ourselves depends, in part, on the words we know. Most of us use only a handful of words to describe our physical experiences. This coloring activity helps you increase your body awareness by expanding your vocabulary of physical sensations. With more descriptive words available, more subtle sensations enter awareness that may not have been apparent before.

---

1. Take a moment to turn inward. Close your eyes, straighten your spine, and place your feet securely on the floor.

2. Become aware of your breath and observe the air moving in and out of your body for a few moments.

3. Scan your body for one to three of the strongest sensations you feel. Now on the opposite page, find the words that best describe those sensations. Add words in the empty spaces if needed. Color in those words using a bold, warm color, such as red or orange.

4. Next, identify one to three subtle sensations in your body. Find the words that best describe these sensations on the next page. Pick a cool color, like green or blue, and color in the words that describe the subtle sensations.

5. Revisit the words you colored in and the sensations they describe. Have your physical sensations changed or remained the same since you started this exercise? What words would you use to describe them now?

6. What is your body trying to tell you through the words you have colored in?

Burning	Pinching	
Cooling	Pressing	
Expanding	Pulling	
Flowing	Softening	
Itching	Tightening	
Numbing	Tingling	
Opening	Vibrating	

EVERY PART OF ME MATTERS.

CONNECTION

IN NATURE'S LAP

PLAYER: 1 | **TIME:** 15 TO 60 MINUTES | **SUPPLIES:** NOTEPAD

Many of us were lucky enough to spend time as children in our grandparents' laps, listening to stories and experiencing what it's like to feel love and belonging. As adults, we can have a similar experience by putting ourselves in nature's lap. Like a beloved grandparent, nature is constantly teaching and telling stories. We just need to take time to sit and listen. When we do, we can reconnect with a sense of awe and appreciation for the ways nature supports us. This journaling activity provides a sense of connection with your surroundings by listening closely to nature's wisdom.

---

1. Choose a place to spend at least 10 minutes outside by yourself. You might prefer to be in the woods or along the shore, but a simple backyard, park, or any other outdoor setting will do just fine.

2. Find a comfortable spot to sit and observe what is happening in nature. Use every sense that is readily available to you: sight, sound, smell, and touch.

3. If your mind drifts (as it probably will), just gently return your awareness to what is present in nature. The following questions can help guide you:

   ◆ What interconnections can you find in nature?

   ◆ What is changing? What is staying the same?

- How much diversity do you observe?

- Where does nature's energy come from?

- What does nature throw away, if anything?

- How does nature solve problems?

- What seems to motivate nature?

4. When you are ready, jot down your insights. How do you feel? What do you want to remember and share with others about this experience?

I IMMERSE MY AWARENESS IN SIMPLE SOUNDS.

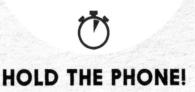

HOLD THE PHONE!

PLAYER: 1 | **TIME:** 5 MINUTES

Technology lets us communicate with just about anyone instantaneously, but it can also make us feel distracted and disconnected from those nearest to us. For many people, technology has become an addiction. We check for social media updates every few minutes. We get lost in long periods of web surfing. Often, we use technology to escape from discomfort or boredom, but we can choose to stay with the uncomfortable experience instead. This quick meditation uses mindful awareness to help you reconnect with yourself and create a healthier relationship with technology.

1. Be on the lookout for an urge to use technology. If you're like most of us, you won't have to wait long!

2. When you feel the urge to grab your smartphone or tablet, pause. Pausing just a moment is great progress. You are bringing awareness to an autopilot process.

3. Now, do the following: Take one deep breath, saying, "With this breath, I see my tech habit wants to launch." On the exhalation, say, "Breathing out, I will choose whether to continue the habit." The importance of this step is to train yourself to see the decision point where you have power.

4. During the next urge, say, "This time, I choose to fully experience the urge before using my phone."

5. Bring direct awareness to your experience of the urge. Start with the physical sensations present in your body. Look for things like tightness in your belly, nervous energy in your chest, or a clenched jaw. Now consider what emotions are present. Do you feel anxiety, anger, or annoyance? Take two minutes to simply feel these uncomfortable feelings.

6. After two minutes, notice how the sensations and emotions have dissipated to some extent. Ask yourself, "Do I still want to use technology as an escape now, or do something else?" It's fine if you still want to use your phone or tablet, of course, but now you have put the decision to do so in your own hands.

WHEN I NEED TO WAIT, I SMILE.

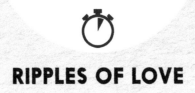

RIPPLES OF LOVE

PLAYER: 1 | **TIME:** 5 TO 10 MINUTES

You've probably seen an image of elegant water ripples. This is a mindfulness favorite, representing the beauty of life's simple moments. Just like a single ripple that can travel very long distances, a loving-kindness meditation generates positive thoughts that can have far-reaching impacts. This exercise uses a simple ancient method to help you cultivate a compassionate mindset. The goal is to gradually expand your compassion to include more and more people.

1. Sit comfortably in an upright position. Center yourself by bringing awareness to your breath for three to four cycles.

2. Offer loving-kindness to yourself by saying the following phrases aloud. Feel free to revise the phrases; just be sure they express unconditional loving-kindness. It's okay if it feels a little forced. The idea is to gradually feel more authentic saying them over time.

May I now be filled with loving-kindness.
May I now be safe and protected.
May I now be resilient in mind and body.
May I now live with ease and joy.

3. Now direct the phrases toward a loved one, like a partner or best friend. Say out loud:

May you now be filled with loving-kindness.
May you now be safe and protected.
May you now be resilient in mind and body.
May you now live with ease and joy.

4. Repeat the phrases for someone you feel neutral toward, like a person you passed on the street or who helped you at a store.

5. Repeat the phrases for someone you feel antagonism toward, such as a colleague you dislike or a politician who aggravates you.

6. Finally, repeat the phrases for everyone on Earth, all plants and animals, all landforms and waterways, all planets, stars, and the entire universe:

May we now be filled with loving-kindness.
May we now be safe and protected.
May we now be resilient in mind and body.
May we now live with ease and joy.

BREATHING IN NOURISHING LIGHT, I BREATHE OUT DISCOMFORT AND UNEASE.

RETHINKING JUDGMENT

PLAYER: 1 | **TIME:** 5 MINUTES

The brain interprets everything we see, hear, touch, taste, smell, think, and feel. The problem is those interpretations are often taken as fact. Say a colleague is late for a meeting. One person thinks, "They don't take this meeting seriously," while another thinks, "They must be having a rough morning." Both interpretations can seem like truth to the thinkers, but the only thing they know for a fact is that the colleague was late. Mistaking interpretation for truth can lead to judgment and miscommunication. Inspired by the book *The 15 Commitments of Conscious Leadership*, this short exercise brings awareness to your interpretations so you can release judgment and avoid miscommunication.

---

1. Identify a situation in which you are being judgmental of someone.

2. Summarize your perspective with the phrase, "I feel *(fill in the blank)* toward *(fill in the blank)* because they did *(fill in the blank)*."

3. Consider what about your perspective is a fact versus an interpretation or judgment. The facts can be observed by any third party. The judgments are how you make meaning by interpreting the facts.

4. Imagine you're with the person you're feeling judgmental toward. Use the "I" statement to describe your internal experience of the situation. For example, you can describe physical sensations: "When you came in late for the meeting, I noticed my stomach churn" or "I noticed my breath get shallow." Or you might describe your emotional reaction: "When you came in late for the meeting, I became nervous" or "I was sympathetic." This way of communicating is effective because no one can question the truth of your internal experience (although it assumes you're being honest with yourself!).

5. Now, try to describe any thoughts or judgments that arose: for example, "I had a story in my head that you don't care about this group," "Judgmental thoughts arose when you came in late," or "I had a thought that you were having a hard start to the day."

➡ **TIP:** Practicing this on your own can make it feel more natural the next time you notice you are jumping to conclusions or judgments toward another person.

WHEN I LISTEN, MY BODY SHARES IMPORTANT INFORMATION.

YOUR KEY CONNECTIONS

PLAYER: 1 | **TIME:** 5 TO 10 MINUTES

Sunlight is an energy source. Photosynthesis transforms sunlight so it can be used by living organisms. As Kathy Allen proposes in *Leading from the Roots*, this is great a metaphor for our life purpose. Think of our sense of purpose as an energy source, like the sun. What is needed to transform our sense of purpose into something useful? One answer is relationships. When we connect with others, we discover where our gifts are needed and how we can contribute to outcomes we could not accomplish alone. This visualization helps deepen your awareness and appreciation for the connecting relationships that help you manifest your life purpose.

---

1. Find a comfortable place to lie down. Relax with a few deep breaths.

2. Think back to five years ago: Hold old were you? Where were you living? What were you doing? What goals did you have? What did you see as your life purpose?

3. Now visualize yourself moving forward in time. Think of the major events and milestones. What happened that helped you know you were on the right track? What setbacks or corrections stand out?

4. As you move forward in time, make special note of the people who were instrumental along the way. Who supported you? Who taught you important lessons? Who pointed the way when you were uncertain? Say their names aloud when you think of them. Each time you think of someone new, try to repeat the other names first before naming that person aloud.

5. Continue moving forward in time until you arrive in the present moment. Say a few words of thanks to each person who helped you reach this point.

6. Now visualize moving forward in time until you reach one year into the future. What do you hope to be doing then? What goals do you have for the coming year? Who might help you manifest your life purpose in the coming months?

I FEEL MY FEELINGS COMPLETELY.

THE ART OF CONVERSATION

PLAYERS: 2 OR MORE | **TIME:** 10 TO 30 MINUTES

A good conversation can create powerful connection. It lets us share our life experiences and gain new understanding. We can provide support by listening deeply. We come up with ideas that would not have occurred to us alone. But some conversations feel like debates, where there's no real personal connection. It's more like speaking at each other rather than talking with each other. Mindful conversations—which have a clear purpose and process—can enrich the quality of connection, develop shared understanding, and set the stage for creating new ideas, too. Use this simple activity to guide your next conversation in a mindful way.

---

1. Sit comfortably, facing each other. Take a few deep breaths to feel grounded. You can set the mood by listening to a brief guided meditation or reading a poem about connection, which you can find with an internet search.

2. Agree on intentions with your conversation partner(s). What is the overall topic? What do you hope to accomplish through the conversation? How do you hope to feel?

3. Then spend a few minutes having a conversation focusing only on facts. For example, if the topic is about climate change, discuss what most people agree are facts about that topic. Agree to gently redirect one another if you notice that you're moving away from facts (just like redirecting your awareness to the breath when your mind wanders in meditation).

4. Now spend a few minutes sharing emotions related to the topic. Do you generally feel positive or negative about this subject? What specific feelings came up for each person? Gently redirect one another if you notice that you're moving away from emotions during this step.

5. Now explore insights. Why is this topic important at this time? What creative solutions might address the issue? What would it take to change the status quo? What difference would that make?

6. Finally, consider action steps. What options do you have for moving this topic forward? Are there actions you want to commit to taking? Who will do what and by when?

I AM THE SOURCE OF MY OWN SAFETY AND APPROVAL.

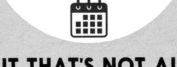

BUT THAT'S NOT ALL!

PLAYERS: 2 OR MORE | **TIME:** 8 TO 10 MINUTES

Many spiritual traditions teach that everything is interconnected. Science supports this, too. Humans need oxygen made by trees. Plants turn sunlight into food that countless organisms rely on. All life is linked to particular physical, chemical, and biological conditions that are needed for survival. Buddhist teacher Thich Nhat Hanh calls this "interbeing." He explains how everything can be found in a piece of paper. A cloud is needed for rain, which is needed to grow trees, which are needed to make pulp. Take away any linkage, and there's no paper. This playful exercise helps you develop this same awareness of interconnection.

---

1. Sit comfortably, facing each other.

2. The first player looks at a simple object and says, "I see a *(fill in the blank)* before me, but that's not all there is." For example, "I see a chair before me, but that's not all there is."

3. The second player links the object to something that caused or supported its existence. For example, "I can see the chair, and I can also see the carpenter who made the chair."

4. The third player (or repeat the first player) adds another linkage, such as "I can see the chair, the carpenter, and also the oatmeal the carpenter had for breakfast."

5. This continues with each player restating the sequence of linkages and adding a new one that builds off the previous one. If a player cannot think of a new linkage, they are out of the game. If a player cannot remember the linkages or states them out of order, they are out of the game.

6. The last player left is the winner. (If no players can think of a new linkage, it's a tie.)

➧ **TIP:** You can increase the difficulty of this game by starting with more challenging objects. For example, instead of a chair, the game could begin with a computer-processing chip.

I TAKE TIME TO CONNECT.

RESCUE FROM A DESERTED ISLAND

PLAYERS: 2 | **TIME:** 10 TO 15 MINUTES

It's easy to isolate ourselves when we are going through a challenging time. We might believe that pushing others away will let us focus on our problem. Or we might feel too vulnerable to allow others a close look at our feelings of uncertainty, regret, or sorrow. Having a mindful two-way conversation about your response to challenges can help you better ask for help and provide support. This activity offers you and a loved one a way to avoid getting stranded on an island.

---

1. Sit comfortably, facing each other.

2. Each player takes a turn sharing an example of a time when they reacted to hardship by retreating to an island. Discuss what motivated your behavior, the effects of the behavior, and what you learned from that life experience.

3. Brainstorm ways you might help each other in future times of uncertainty. Consider these prompts:

   ◆ **The ask.** When suffering, we can feel overwhelmed, confused, and isolated. A prepared script can help. In his book *How to Love*, teacher Thich Nhat Hanh suggests these simple sentences: *My dear, I am suffering. I feel _____ (worried, angry, anxious) and I want you to know it. I am doing my best. Please help me.*

◆ **Potential responses.** When someone asks us for help, we may want to fix the problem or give advice. But often the person simply needs acknowledgment and compassion, such as: (a) Listening without judgment. Simply say, "Tell me all about it." (b) Mirroring back what you heard and asking, "Am I understanding you correctly?" (c) Asking the person to locate somewhere in their body that feels calm and safe, and inviting them to breathe into it.

4. Even with this preparation, it can be difficult to take skillful action in challenging moments. Agree on a simple signal you can use when saying words is too difficult. It may be a particular emoji you can text one another or a gesture like putting your hand over your heart.

5. End your mindful conversation by expressing gratitude to each other for your supportive relationship.

I MAKE ROOM FOR NEW PERSPECTIVES.

THE MINDFUL HEART

PLAYER: 1 | **TIME:** 15 MINUTES | **SUPPLIES:** PENCIL OR PEN

Living an openhearted life means embodying a loving, curious, and accepting presence regardless of the circumstances. Most of us have received this type of love in life, whether from family, friends, or even a pet. Meditation teachers often speak of living this way, too. But what if we get so focused on the mechanics of meditating "correctly" that we miss out on the openhearted part? This activity helps you identify people and pets who have modeled openhearted love in your life. It reminds you that even simple, everyday actions, when done mindfully, can express an open and mindful heart.

---

1. Sit comfortably and take a few breaths to center yourself.

2. Recall times in your life when you felt another's openhearted presence. Allow yourself to go through those memories at your own pace. Try to recall specific scenes, situations, sounds, and smells associated with those times.

3. In the heart on the next page, write the names of those who were part of your openhearted memories. Feel free to color in the heart or doodle around it.

4. Now think about each person (or animal!) whose name you put into the heart. In your mind's eye, imagine where they are today. Think of what they might be doing, what brings them joy, and what worries they may have. If the person or animal is deceased, think of one of their close loved ones who is still with us.

5. Imagine yourself being openhearted toward each person whose name is in your heart. What would you say or do? Where? How would the recipient respond? What would happen afterward? How would you feel?

6. Pick one of these actions to carry out. Who will receive your openhearted presence?

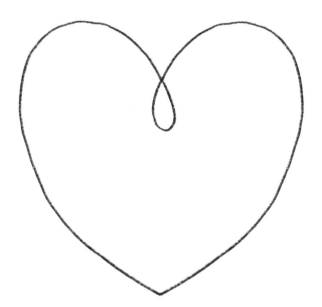

LOVE IS AN ONGOING ACT OF LEARNING.

RESOLVING CONFLICT

PLAYER: 1 | **TIME:** 5 MINUTES

Have you ever been in an argument where both sides dig in their heels? These arguments can be harmful to relationships, whether the topic is big (moving to a new city) or small (what to have for dinner). Many conflicts happen when we stop being open to new solutions. We would rather defend our position than explore other ways to meet our needs. Mindful awareness and communication can minimize such conflicts by helping us be clear about the root causes of our arguments and what we need for resolution. This quick exercise can help you clarify what you really need so you can mindfully communicate it to others.

---

1. Take a moment to set aside distractions. You might turn off your phone, go to a place where you can be alone, and/or light a candle.

2. Recall a recurring disagreement you have with someone. Bring that person's presence into your awareness and offer them a loving-kindness meditation (see "Ripples of Love" on page 72).

3. Now consider the argument: What is wrong and how would you fix it? Say, "The problem is *(fill in the blank)*, and the solution is *(fill in the blank)*!" For example, "The problem is that my partner puts the silverware point-side up in the dishwasher, and when I poke my hand unloading the dishes, they think that's funny. The solution is to put the silverware facing down *and* be more considerate of my feelings!"

4. Consider what your underlying needs might be. What need is at the root of this issue for you? Some examples are *meaning, honesty, autonomy, sustenance, safety, order, belonging, empathy,* and *love.* Choose what resonates most with you right now.

5. Now make a clear request to have your needs met. "I have a need for *(fill in the blank)*. You could meet that need by *(fill in the blank)*. Would you be willing to *(fill in the blank)*?" For example: "I have a need for empathy that is not being met. You could meet this need by showing you care when I get hurt. Will you acknowledge that I'm in pain when the silverware pokes my hand?"

➧ **TIP:** Notice that in the example the underlying issue isn't about the orientation of the silverware. The person needs empathy from their partner. When this is made clear, the discussion can focus on the real issue.

I SET ASIDE TIME TO GET TO KNOW MYSELF.

5

JOY

WHEN THE LIST IS DONE

PLAYER: 1 | **TIME:** 5 MINUTES
SUPPLIES: PEN AND PAPER OR VIRTUAL NOTEPAD

Have you ever wondered what it would feel like to have nothing left on your to-do list? No laundry, no groceries, no errands, no project to finish, no trip to take. Let it sink in: Nothing. To. Do. How would you feel? Does it sound like joyful liberation? We might have this experience on vacation, when the days are more open-ended and the tasks feel less urgent. But what if we don't have to go on vacation or finish our to-do list to feel this way? What if we could create this feeling inside ourselves whenever we want? This satisfying activity can help you do just that!

---

1. Write out a *long* to-do list. Include the things that really weigh you down, like what you *should* do. Also include what you could do if only you had the chance and what you would do if you had the time.

2. Look over the list, feeling the weight of everything that is undone.

3. Now ask yourself, "What would I be without these to-do items? How would I be different?" Write down five to seven words that describe who you would be without the items on your list.

4. Now cross everything off the list you can't do in the next month. (This doesn't mean you will never do them, just that you aren't doing them right now.) Take satisfaction in crossing them off your list. You might make a long, slow, dark line through the middle; draw a big, fat *X* over them; scribble them out; or block them out in black.

5. Now cross off everything you can't do in the coming week. Again, enjoy crossing the items off. This is cross-off therapy!

6. Now cross off everything you can't do in the next day.

7. Now cross off everything you can't do in the next hour.

8. Now cross off everything you can't do in the next minute.

9. You are now in the present moment. What is left on the list?

10. How do you feel? Carry this feeling, which may include openness, relief, and ease, into the next thing you choose to do.

I APPROACH NEW SITUATIONS WITH CURIOSITY.

BENDING TIME WITH JOY

PLAYER: 1 | **TIME:** 5 MINUTES

We think of time as linear. Life marches through minutes, hours, days, and years. There's no going back, right? Maybe it's not so simple. For example, brain research shows that our memories change whenever we remember them. So, although time moves forward, our understanding of the past seems to be less linear. Emotions are another example. We usually believe that "because X happens, I feel Y." But that's not so. We can change our feelings, no matter what happens in "real time." Feelings from the past can be brought forward. It just takes a little practice. Try this visualization to mindfully shift neutral or negative emotions toward joy.

1. Sit in a comfortable position. Place your hands palms down on top of your legs: left hand on your left leg, right hand on your right leg.

2. Identify what you are feeling in the present moment. Then decide how strong that feeling is on a scale of 1 (weak) to 10 (very strong). You might say, "I'm feeling frustrated at level six."

3. Now think of a time you felt joyful. Be specific. How old were you? What were you doing? Were others present or were you alone?

4. Recall the joyful feeling from your memory. Invite that feeling into the present moment. Begin to re-create it in your body.

5. Now imagine yourself in a bubble surrounded by the feeling of joy you experienced.

6. Begin alternately tapping your legs with your hands in a steady, even pace: left-right, left-right. Continue imagining yourself in the joy bubble while you tap for two to three minutes.

7. As you tap, use these questions to reconnect with your experience of joy:

➡ What color is the joy bubble you're in? What is the temperature? What sounds fill the bubble of joy?

➡ What physical sensations do you experience?

➡ What kinds of thoughts do you have inside the joy bubble?

8. When you're ready, gradually let the tapping come to a natural end. Take a deep breath. Notice how you feel now.

I ABIDE IN WHAT'S HERE, NOW.

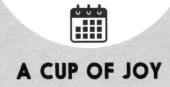

A CUP OF JOY

PLAYER: 1 | **TIME:** 5 TO 10 MINUTES
SUPPLIES: YOUR FAVORITE MORNING DRINK

It's easy to spend your entire life waiting for the next best thing. As teens, we can't wait to become adults. Then we wait for jobs we like. Then it's waiting to have enough money for a home or family. Along the way, we wait for promotions, vacations, the right relationships, and other milestones. The only people who seem to not be waiting are young children, who are better able to abide in the present moment. And they seem to have more fun, too! With mindfulness, we don't need to wait for joyful experiences because they're available to us all the time. This simple activity is about creating joy in everyday activities.

---

1. Prepare to make your favorite morning drink, such as coffee, tea, or a smoothie.

2. Arrange the ingredients on your countertop. Take great care as if you're displaying them for an esteemed guest.

3. Moving at a gentle pace, notice small, sensory details, such as the curve and temperature of your cup and the distribution of a spoon's weight in your hand.

4. Begin preparing the drink. Note the sounds of liquid pouring into metal, glass, or earthenware. Pay attention to every texture you touch. Inhale the aromas of your tea bag, coffee grounds, or other ingredients.

5. Once your drink is ready, sit down and set the drink in front of you. Look at the shadows cast across your cup or glass. Notice the colors of the liquid, the cup, and the table. Observe the liquid's surface—are there bubbles or movement? Is it creamy or translucent?

6. Close your eyes. Spend a minute smelling your drink. Switch between actively inhaling the aroma and passively allowing the scent to drift into your nostrils. Feel the temperature of your drink as you hover above it.

7. Take a sip. Immerse yourself in the sensations: the heat or cold, how it feels across your tongue and going down your throat, and the flavor it leaves in your mouth.

8. Continue to enjoy your drink with mindfulness. Notice the heightened sensations. Appreciate the joy that comes from nurturing these simple sensory pleasures.

I PRACTICE "ENOUGHNESS."

FINDING JOY IN NATURE

PLAYER: 1 | **TIME:** 15 TO 20 MINUTES

Nature certainly looks joyful at times. The excited smile of a puppy, a beautiful sunrise, the acrobatic glee of dolphins, and colorful springtime flowers all look like happy celebrations. Whether or not nature itself experiences joy, it can bring out our joyful qualities. Researchers have found that spending time in nature can increase happiness, kindness, connectedness, and creativity. This fun meditation taps your imaginative curiosity to discover and experience joy in nature. If "looking" for joy feels forced at first, it's okay. Simply calling to mind positive qualities like joy can have real benefits, even if they're not arising on their own.

---

1. Find an area outside where you can explore at a calm, meandering pace, like a park, campground, or hiking trail.

2. Begin by looking for joy in the smallest things. For example, are there tiny insects whose colors or patterns seem exuberant to you? Or a twig that's proudly mimicking a giant tree? Or a tiny burst of pink petal that's fallen from a flower?

3. Next, look for joy among things that live close to the ground, like playful rabbits, precocious chipmunks, and vibrant shrubs. Which plants seem especially happy to be alive? Do any of the rocks appear to be smiling?

4. Now look at living things you find at a level approximately between your knees and the highest you can reach. This may include smaller tree species with jubilant flowers or cheerily outstretched branches. You may see the bursting yellow of finches at a bird feeder, or tall flowering grasses displaying delightful seedpods.

5. Turn your awareness upward now, from treetops to the farthest reaches of sky. Is there bliss in the way light passes through branches? Can you see joy in the shapes of clouds or the pureness of color that reaches to the atmosphere's edge?

6. Finally, look for joyful patterns that repeat across all these scales, from tiny to expansive. Where do you see symmetrical spirals, waves, stripes, or repeating shapes? Enjoy the abundance of the living things all around, beautifully designed to thrive in their ecological niche.

I RELEASE WHAT DOES NOT SERVE ME.

TIME-TRAVELING JOY

PLAYER: 1 | **TIME:** 5 MINUTES

This quick activity is for when you don't feel joyful. Maybe you got disappointing news, are discouraged by a project, or even just had a poor night's sleep. Whether you're crabby, sad, worried, or down in the dumps, it's all welcome here. But beware: Negative energy multiplies. One worry leads to another. The mind conjures worst-case scenarios as it revisits old gripes and criticizes imperfections. Quick! Use this guide to teleport yourself back in time and then return to present-moment joy.

1. Sit up straight, place your feet securely on the floor, and put your hands on your knees. Take three to four deep breaths, moving your awareness to your belly as it expands and contracts. Relax.

2. Now recall a time in life when you felt genuinely joyful. It could be a memory from last week or from your youth. That you felt joy and know it was the real thing are the only criteria.

3. Revisit the details of that time. Who was present? How did they contribute to the joyful experience? What happened? What was the joy-filled "plot" of the situation?

4. Slowly scan your mind for specific visual memories. See if new ones emerge that you haven't thought of in a while. Recall the sounds and smells as best as you can.

5. Use your memory and intention to re-create joyful sensations like tingling arms, warmth in the face, openness in the chest, or any other physical sensations from that time. Make the facial expressions you made during the experience, and give voice to the sounds you made, whether words, laughter, or hoots.

6. Now sustain the joyful sensations you have generated but allow the memory to recede. You just time traveled—and returned with the gift of your own joy!

I ADVOCATE FOR MY WELL-BEING.

HOW MANY YOUS?

PLAYER: 1 | **TIME:** 5 MINUTES

We take a lot for granted. Our body breathes on its own, and air is freely available. So much goes into generating the electricity we use, the water we drink, and even the hobbies we love. We benefit greatly from others' efforts, both present and past. When we broaden our perspective to include everything behind the scenes that makes our lives possible, our everyday worries seem less important. This perspective-broadening exercise was inspired by an interactive online graphic called "The Scale of the Universe 2." It illuminates how our daily concerns are nested within a larger unfolding of phenomena, which can spark appreciation, wonder, and joy.

1. Lie down in a comfortable place. Feel the warmth of your breath and the aliveness of your body.

2. Notice the space you occupy. About how many of you would it take to reach across the room? How about to the ceiling?

3. Now consider your position relative to others: Approximately 20 of your body lengths equals the length of an average blue whale. Imagine coming across one of those!

4. Now imagine a redwood tree. About 50 of you would reach a redwood's highest point.

5. The top of Mount Everest equals about 4,800 of you. You could start your own town! That seems like a lot, but if you're a runner, you go 23,000 lengths-of-you when you run a marathon. And to span the Grand Canyon? 244,000. Picture that!

6. Now imagine a hummingbird. It would take about 18.5 hummingbirds from end to end to equal your height. It would take 34 chicken eggs, 380 grains of rice, and 3,800 grains of salt. Can you imagine those lying end to end alongside you?

7. A mote of dust is about the smallest thing the naked human eye can see. It would take 6,500 motes of dust to reach your height.

8. Zoom in even more. Imagine how many molecules make up your body. More than a septillion! Think about the atoms, too, in those molecules.

9. Did you notice a shift in perspective? How does this affect your sense of scale? Become attuned with the awesome mystery of our universe and your place in it.

I CONNECT WITH MY PURPOSE.

QUICK COMPLIMENTS

PLAYERS: 2 | **TIME:** 5 MINUTES | **SUPPLIES:** TIMER

Positive feedback at home and work fosters appreciation and abundance. It develops reciprocity and loyalty. It contributes to trusting relationships, which support our best thinking, doing, and being. Research shows that five positive comments for every negative one results in the most flourishing relationships. Unfortunately, most of us stink at giving positive feedback! This "lightning round" game helps you practice giving meaningful, positive feedback to others spontaneously and mindfully.

1. Sit comfortably facing each other and set the timer for three minutes.

2. Take turns expressing joyful appreciation for each other until the timer goes off.

3. To add another dimension to this game, track score of the feedback based on its type.

   ◆ **Appearance (1 point):** surface-level appreciations, such as "I like your haircut" or "I dig your shirt." These can help build momentum early in the game, but push yourself to go deeper!

   ◆ **Action (3 points):** feedback that focuses on things the other person does, such as "I am fond of your cooking" or "I like that you are usually on time."

- **Qualities (5 points):** comments that reveal the other person's qualities, such as "I enjoy your sense of humor" or "I adore your sensitivity toward others."

- **Appreciation (10 points):** affirmations that connect action, response, and insight. Use the formula, "When you *(fill in the blank)*, I feel *(fill in the blank)*. I appreciate your ability to meet my need for *(fill in the blank)*. Thank you." Here's an example of this formula with a loved one: "When you gently ask why I'm being quiet, I feel cared for. I appreciate your ability to meet my need to be seen and understood. Thank you." Here's an example in the workplace: "When you take responsibility for your part of the situation, I feel respect for you. I appreciate your ability to meet my need for accountability. Thank you."

4. Tally your scores and spend one to two minutes discussing what stands out about the experience.

I LET ALL LIFE'S ENERGY MOVE THROUGH ME.

LAUGHING MEDITATION

PLAYERS: 2 OR MORE | **TIME:** 5 MINUTES | **SUPPLIES:** TIMER

Sometimes mindfulness can seem like serious business. However, many Buddhist masters are known for their childlike openness, big smiles, and playful wit. Included among them is His Holiness the 14th Dalai Lama, who believes that humor and openness are important parts of mindfulness practice. In fact, laughter has many benefits: It boosts the immune system, lowers stress, and burns calories. It also enhances teamwork. Amazingly, studies have shown that even fake laughter can generate the same benefits. This activity will help you deepen mindful awareness through play, humor, and spontaneity.

1. All players stand up and mentally note how they are feeling. How would they describe their body sensations? How would they rate their level of energy on a scale of 1 to 10 (where 1 is sluggish and 10 is energized)? There's no need to share this aloud; just take note.

2. Set the timer for three minutes. Now, everyone starts laughing, faking it as necessary, until the timer goes off. Everyone should have a really good belly laugh.

3. Once you catch your breath, players can share how they feel. Here are some questions to guide you:

➡ What did you notice during this experience?

➡ Did your score on the scale change?

➡ What will be different now as you all carry on with your day?

➡ **TIP:** Try this activity virtually during a video chat or virtual meeting. Just make sure everyone turns on their sound!

I CHANNEL MY PASSION INTO SERVICE TO THE WORLD.

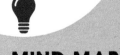

JOYFUL MIND MAP

PLAYER: 1 | **TIME:** 10 TO 15 MINUTES
SUPPLIES: COLORED PENCILS, MARKERS, OR CRAYONS

A mind map is a diagram that links together parts of a whole, often using circled words or phrases to show the relationship between them. Mind maps are not only great for discovering connections, brainstorming solutions, and exploring new ways of thinking, they're also fun to draw! By creating a mind map of who and what you appreciate, you can bring your awareness to things that are going well and that bring you joy. This results in a more optimistic outlook, which has numerous physical and psychological benefits. This creative activity helps you put a mindful focus on the positive aspects of your life.

---

1. On the next page, write your name in the center circle.

2. In the two circles connected to the center circle, write the names of people who make a positive impact in your day-to-day life.

3. Draw two additional circles using any color. Write the names of places you regularly go that you appreciate—perhaps a café, park, movie theater, or even a favorite chair.

4. Next, draw two circles with another color and write specific experiences that you enjoy. Again, anything goes—for example, going for a walk, taking a nap, reading your favorite books, listening to music, or even certain times of day! Reflect on what you enjoy doing and add it to your map.

5. Using a new color, draw lines linking the people, places, and experiences that are already connected. For example, if you go for walks with your mom at the park, connect all those circles.

6. Next, use another color showing potential connections. Perhaps you could go to a new place with an old friend or introduce them to an activity you normally do with others?

7. Lastly, use a final color or a dotted line showing potential connections for others. Are there people in your life who might enjoy knowing one another? Could you recommend certain places or activities that others might appreciate as much as you do?

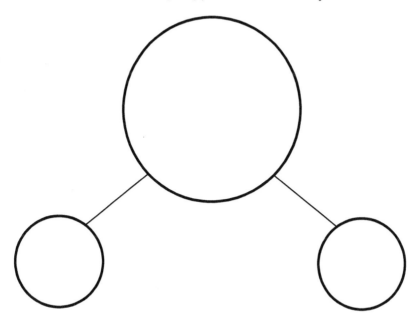

CHOOSING JOY

PLAYER: 1 | **TIME:** 10 TO 15 MINUTES |
SUPPLIES: COLORED PENCILS, MARKERS, OR CRAYONS

Sometimes it may seem like a sense of well-being is not within our control. This is because we often feel subject to the thoughts and emotions we experience. Life appears to happen to us, compelled by outside forces. With mindfulness, we realize that we have choices. We can't stop thoughts or challenging emotions from happening, but we can choose our responses. We can also nurture positive mental states rather than negative ones. This coloring activity helps you recognize joy in everyday moments, which will help you respond more calmly to difficult emotions when they happen.

---

1. Your task is to find joy in nine things where you have never seen it before.

2. Begin by examining the objects in your immediate vicinity. For example, the assorted, everyday objects on your desk. Pick up an object and look for a quality that offers you a small dose of delight.

3. When you identify a joyful quality, write it in one of the nine circles on the opposite page. Here are some examples:

   ◆ The smoothness of a lip balm container.

   ◆ The crinkling sound of a plastic bag.

   ◆ The precision of a smartphone design.

   ◆ The cool breeze created by flipping a book's pages near your cheek.

4. Then pick up another object and do the same thing. Continue until all nine circles have a joyful quality written in them. (You may need to get objects from around the room if there aren't nine within arm's reach.)

5. Color in your circles, choosing whatever colors bring you the most joy!

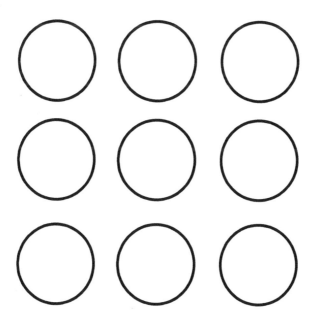

I DESERVE LOVE.

Resources

BOOKS

Brach, Tara, PhD. *True Refuge: Finding Peace and Freedom in Your Own Awakened Heart.* Bantam Books, 2013.

Chödrön, Pema. *Getting Unstuck: Breaking Your Habitual Patterns and Encountering Naked Reality.* Sounds True, 2005.

Dethmer, Jim, Diana Chapman, and Kaley Warner Klemp. *The 15 Commitments of Conscious Leadership: A New Paradigm for Sustainable Success.* The Conscious Leadership Group, 2015.

Hanh, Thich Nhat. *Being Peace.* Parallax Press, 1987.

Hanh, Thich Nhat. *How to Love.* Parallax Press, 2015.

Kabat-Zinnm Jon. *Full Catastrophe Living: Using the Wisdom of Your Body and Mind to Face Stress, Pain, and Illness.* Bantam Books, 2013.

Kelly, Loch. *The Way of Effortless Mindfulness: A Revolutionary Guide for Living an Awakened Life.* Sounds True, 2019. Audiobook.

Kornfield, Jack. *After the Ecstasy, the Laundry: How the Heart Grows Wise on the Spiritual Path.* Bantam Books, 2000.

Peat, F. David. *Gentle Action: Bringing Creative Change to a Turbulent World.* Pari Publishing, 2008.

Singer, Michael A. *The Untethered Soul: The Journey Beyond Yourself.* New Harbinger Publications, 2007.

Treleaven, David A. *Trauma-Sensitive Mindfulness: Practices for Safe and Transformative Healing.* W. W. Norton & Company, 2018.

Whyte, David. *When the Heart Breaks: A Journey Through Requited and Unrequited Love.* Sounds True, 2013. Audiobook.

WEBSITES

Conscious Leadership Group: Conscious.is

Palouse Mindfulness: PalouseMindfulness.com

PODCASTS

On Being with Krista Tippett (OnBeing.org/series/podcast)

APPS

Insight Timer: InsightTimer.com

Mindleap: Mindleap.com

Waking Up with Sam Harris: WakingUp.com

References

Adams, A. J. "Seeing Is Believing: The Power of Visualization."
Psychology Today. December 3, 2009. PsychologyToday.com/us
/blog/flourish/200912/seeing-is-believing-the-power-visualization.

Allen, Dr. Kathleen E. *Leading from the Roots: Nature-Inspired
Leadership Lessons for Today's World.* New York: Morgan James
Publishing, 2018.

Boynton, Emily. "How Meditation Affects Your Brain and Boosts
Well-Being." Right as Rain by UW Medicine. October 26, 2020.
RightAsRain.uwmedicine.org/mind/well-being/science-behind
-meditation.

Centers for Disease Control and Prevention. "Physical Activity
Breaks for the Workplace: Resource Guide." CDC.gov. May 2021.
CDC.gov/workplacehealthpromotion/initiatives/resource-center
/pdf/Workplace-Physical-Activity-Break-Guide-508.pdf.

Dethmer, Jim, Diana Chapman, and Kaley Warner Klemp. *The
15 Commitments of Conscious Leadership: A New Paradigm for
Sustainable Success.* The Conscious Leadership Group, 2014.

Goodnet. "Head, Heart, and Gut: How to Use the 3 Brains." August 20,
2020. Goodnet.org/articles/head-heart-gut-how-to-use-3-brains.

Guy-Evans, Olivia. "Parasympathetic Nervous System Functions."
SimplyPsychology. May 18, 2021. SimplyPsychology.org
/parasympathetic-nervous-system.html.

Halifax, Joan. *Being with Dying: Cultivating Compassion and Fear-
lessness in the Presence of Death.* Boulder, CO: Shambhala, 2008.

Hanh, Thich Nhat. *How to Love*. Berkeley, CA: Parallax Press, 2015.

Hanh, Thich Nhat. *Peace Is Every Step: The Path of Mindfulness in Everyday Life*. New York: Bantam Books, 1991.

Hanh, Thich Nhat. *Present Moment Wonderful Moment: Mindfulness Verses for Daily Living*. 2nd ed. Berkeley, CA: Parallax Press, 2006.

Huang, Cary. "The Scale of the Universe 2." Accessed August 12, 2021. HTwins.net/scale2.

Jump Start by WebMD. "Why Sitting Too Much Is Bad for Your Health." Accessed August 12, 2021. WebMD.com/fitness-exercise /ss/slideshow-sitting-health.

Kelly, Loch. *Shift into Freedom: The Science and Practice of Open-Hearted Awareness*. Boulder, CO: Sounds True, 2015.

Matta, Christy. "Posture and How It Changes Your Feelings." MentalHelp.net: An American Addiction Centers Resource. Accessed August 16, 2021. MentalHelp.net/blogs/posture-and -how-it-changes-your-feelings.

McNaney, Jenna. "5 Benefits We Can Reap from the Power of Visu- alization Immediately." *HuffPost* blog. Last modified April 14, 2015. HuffPost.com/entry/5-benefits-we-can-reap-fr_b_6672638.

Medical Xpress. "Brain Represents Tools as Temporary Body Parts, Study Confirms." June 22, 2009. MedicalXpress.com/news/2009 -06-brain-tools-temporary-body.html.

Mindful Staff. "Jon Kabat-Zinn: Defining Mindfulness." *Mindful*. January 11, 2017. Mindful.org/jon-kabat-zinn-defining-mindfulness.

Mindful Staff. "The Science of Mindfulness." *Mindful*. September 7, 2020. Mindful.org/the-science-of-mindfulness.

Mindful Staff. "What Is Mindfulness?" *Mindful.* July 8, 2020. Mindful
.org/what-is-mindfulness.

Nguyen, Thai. "Total Number of Synapses in the Adult Human
Neocortex." *Undergraduate Journal of Mathematical Modeling:
One + Two* 3, no. 1 (2010). dx.doi.org/10.5038/2326-3652.3.1.26.

Ostaseski, Frank. *The Five Invitations: Discovering What Death Can
Teach Us About Living Fully.* New York: Flatiron Books, 2017.

Robinson, Lawrence, Melinda Smith, and Jeanne Segal. "Laughter
Is the Best Medicine." HelpGuide. Last modified July 2021.
HelpGuide.org/articles/mental-health/laughter-is-the-best
-medicine.htm#.

Schulkin, Jay, and Greta B. Raglan. "The Evolution of Music and
Human Social Capability." *Frontiers in Neuroscience* 8 (September
17, 2014): 292. doi.org/10.3389/fnins.2014.00292.

Schwartz, Richard C., and Martha Sweezy. *Internal Family Systems
Therapy.* 2nd ed. New York: The Guilford Press, 2019.

Siegel, Daniel J. *The Developing Mind: Toward a Neurobiology of
Interpersonal Experience.* New York: The Guilford Press, 1999.

Smith, Emily Esfahani. "The Benefits of Optimism Are Real." *The
Atlantic.* March 1, 2013. TheAtlantic.com/health/archive/2013/03
/the-benefits-of-optimism-are-real/273306.

Suttie, Jill. "How Nature Can Make You Kinder, Happier, and More
Creative." *Greater Good Magazine.* March 2, 2016. GreaterGood
.berkeley.edu/article/item/how_nature_makes_you_kinder
_happier_more_creative.

Treleaven, David A. *Trauma-Sensitive Mindfulness: Practices for Safe
and Transformative Healing.* W. W. Norton & Company, 2018.

Watkins, Thayer. "Animal Longevity and Scale." San José State University. Accessed August 12, 2021. SJSU.edu/faculty/watkins/longevity.htm.

Zenger, Jack, and Joseph Folkman. "The Ideal Praise-to-Criticism Ratio." *Harvard Business Review*. March 15, 2013. HBR.org/2013/03/the-ideal-praise-to-criticism.

Acknowledgments

I would like to thank all those who have dedicated their lives to cultivating mindfulness and helping others learn to do the same. I am especially grateful to those who have guided my inner journey through their teachings and examples, including Loch Kelly, Thich Nhat Hanh, Pema Chödrön, Jack Kornfield, Jon Kabat-Zinn, Richard Schwartz, Steven Bowman, Ann-Marie McKelvey, the faculty and students at the Mindfulness Coaching School, the Conscious Leadership Group, the Clouds in Water Zen Center, and the Effortless Mindfulness online community. Thank you to Emma, Megan, Annie, and Kate for your care, presence, conversation, and love. Thank you to Annie Choi and Carol Killman Rosenberg for your kind and direct editorial skills and to everyone at Callisto Media who has contributed to making this book possible. Finally, thank you to every wise soul with the foresight to use joy and play to create positive change.
    And thanks, Mom.

About the Author

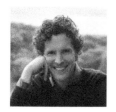

Matthew Rezac is an online mindfulness-based coach who helps clients unravel limiting habits to reveal their innate courage, calm, and creativity. A certified meditation teacher, Matt has explored many traditions, including Vipassana, Zen, and Tibetan Buddhism. In recent years, he's focused on "effortless mindfulness" via meditation teacher Loch Kelly. Matt teaches the Art of Engaged Mindfulness at the Mindfulness Coaching School. Learn more at MatthewRezac.com.